Paleo Diet Plan

How to Start Autoimmune Paleo?

7 Day Autoimmune Paleo Diet Plan- Change Your Diet to Heal Your Body

Table of Contents

Introduction

I would like to thank and congratulate you for buying the book Paleo Diet Plan: How to Start Autoimmune Paleo? 7 Day Autoimmune Paleo Diet Plan- Change Your Diet to Heal Your Body.

This book teaches us the basics of the autoimmune paleo protocol diet or AIP and provides a week-long sample meal plan based on the AIP food list. Useful tips, recipes and guidelines will help readers view the AIP diet as a major lifestyle change that can become therapeutic for the gut, which has become the cradle of debilitating autoimmune conditions.

In a nutshell, autoimmune disease is a state wherein the body's immune system attacks itself and damages the lining of the intestines, thus allowing the passage of harmful bacteria and toxins. Vital organs and blood cells are damaged as a result of this self-attacking disorder.

Though science may claim that this debilitating disease is passed on through genetics, some studies have proven that problems within the immune system are a result of unhealthy habits involving daily activities such as exercise, sleep and nutrition.

This material will help us on our journey towards repairing our digestive tract and preventing autoimmune disease from taking over our lives. Moreover, with the AIP meal planning method, we can create long-term positive effects to our health by simply changing our food choices.

Thanks again for buying this book, I hope you enjoy it!

Chapter 1: Autoimmune Paleo Diet 101: How Food Choices Affect the Body

"The doctor of the future will no longer treat the human frame with drugs, but rather will cure and prevent disease with nutrition."

Thomas Edison

One out of five people suffer from autoimmune disease symptoms which began from simple food sensitivities. Constant digestion of processed food and gut-reactive ingredients such as gluten, sugar and spices lead to food intolerance, hormonal imbalance and abrupt movements in blood and cholesterol levels. These unpleasant factors subsequently cause the immune system to function abnormally.

Luckily, Paleolithic diet advocates which include nutritionists and other health professionals have developed a restrictive yet healthier eating plan that aims to help autoimmune disease sufferers cope with agonizing symptoms and potentially experience remission. This life-changing diet is called the autoimmune paleo protocol diet, which is also known as the AIP diet.

Before we dwell on the guidelines of the AIP diet, let us explore the relationship between autoimmunity and nutrition. This will help us realize how essential it is to choose organic produce for daily meal preparation.

What Is an Autoimmune Disease?

The term *autoimmune* combines two words, *auto* and *immune*, that help explain the basics of this debilitating disease. While a healthy immune system has antibodies that are able to distinguish the good from the harmful bacteria, the antibodies of a person suffering from autoimmune disease instantly attacks all organisms it comes in contact with, including healthy tissue cells.

With autoimmune disease, antibodies mistakenly attack healthy tissue in the intestinal wall because it sees it as a threat. The aftermath of tissue damage is cell inflammation which leads to autoimmune disease, organ damage and unpleasant physical symptoms such as allergies, aches and over-fatigue. In most cases, uncontrolled autoimmune conditions result to death.

There are over 80 autoimmune diseases affecting people all over the world and this has lead to the creation of pharmaceuticals that help control the triggers of the disease. However, a more effective approach towards healing an autoimmune condition is to take medicines and supplements while observing food restrictions. This formula will help detoxify the stomach and rebuild damaged cell walls.

The Link between Food and Autoimmune Disease

A person with an autoimmune disease needs to nourish himself with organic foods to help lessen symptoms and restore normal antibody function in the intestines. Though medical research has claimed that autoimmunity is genetically transferred, recent studies have shown that unhealthy food choices are the culprits of a leaky gut, which is known as a starting point of autoimmune disease.

It is common knowledge that eating unhealthy, processed foods on a regular basis leads to gut problems and hormonal imbalance, which subsequently messes up the normal activity of the immune system. Once the immune system reacts differently and starts attacking the cells it was supposed to protect, disease is introduced into the body.

To manage the triggers of autoimmune disease, doctors recommend avoiding processed dishes, sugar, grains, beans, dairy, nightshade vegetables, alcohol and other harmful ingredients that are not included in a basic Paleolithic diet. Feasting on healthy organic produce such as fruits, vegetables, meat, fatty fish and healthy oils is the best way to heal our body's cells.

The correlation between food and autoimmune disease is the reason why doctors and nutritionists has developed an advanced version of the typical caveman diet and called it the autoimmune paleo protocol diet, or AIP. This has helped a lot of individuals manage the symptoms of their chronic illness and live a more comfortable life.

Benefits of the Autoimmune Paleo Diet

The AIP diet originated from the conventional Paleolithic diet, though it has more food restrictions and lesser room for error. An AIP food list is provided and needs to be strictly followed in order to reap the benefits of its therapeutic properties.

Advocates of the AIP diet have experienced significant transformations as a result of healthier meals. In fact, the following autoimmune conditions can be placed in remission by adopting Paleolithic eating habits:

- Eczema
- Psoriasis
- Rheumatoid arthritis
- Lupus
- Type 1 Diabetes
- Vitiligo
- Crohn's Disease
- Multiple sclerosis
- Celiac disease
- Hashimoto's Disease

Nevertheless, this healthy diet plan is not a miracle cure for autoimmune disease sufferers since doctor-prescribed pharmaceuticals should still be taken regularly. However, creating a meal plan around the AIP food list can greatly help in healing damaged tissues and lessening inflammation all over the body.

The food items in the AIP diet contain high doses of omega-3, potassium, beta carotene, fiber, iron, Vitamin D and Vitamin C. Moreover, the food list is tailor-fit for people who are suffering from immunity-related problems because it teaches them to become creative with cleaner and healthier ingredients.

Apart from food, supplements play a huge role in healing the intestinal wall. The following supplements go hand-in-hand with AIP-friendly foods in helping repair damaged gut tissue:

- L-glutamine
- Multivitamins
- Magnesium
- Probiotic supplements
- Collagen
- Pancreatin
- Cod Liver Oil

Normally, AIP diet specialists recommend 6 to 8 weeks of strictly following the plan's food list if you have an autoimmunity problem. However, people who are not suffering from autoimmune disease but are seeing early symptoms can try out this special diet for 30 days.

After the initial 30-day period, it is acceptable to reintroduce other paleo-friendly foods listed on the succeeding chapter to determine food sensitivities and allow a bit of leeway when it comes to meal preparation. However, if you suffer from full blown autoimmune disease, it is a must to follow the AIP diet permanently until a full recovery has been determined.

No matter how difficult the AIP diet may seem, it really is worth trying if your focus is on healing the body with food. Creating an AIP diet meal plan and stocking the kitchen with AIP-friendly ingredients will help kick start your journey towards optimal wellness.

The succeeding chapters will show a comprehensive autoimmune paleo diet food list as well as one week's worth of delicious recipes that you can cook in your own kitchen. A remarkable change in eating habits can go a long way in determining a healthy and pain-free existence for you and the whole family.

Chapter 2: Autoimmune Paleo Diet Food List

If you are willing to heal your body by embracing the autoimmune paleo diet, then you have just made the best decision of your life. Not only will the AIP diet nourish your body with healthy doses of vitamins and minerals, it will even let you savor the aromatic flavors and textures of clean, gut-friendly natural produce.

The colorful array of fruits, vegetables, meats, herbs and oils will satisfy your taste buds and soothe your stomach. Here is the AIP diet food list which will serve as your basis for healthy meal planning:

Foods allowed in the AIP diet:
Vegetables – artichoke, green onions, avocado, beets, broccoli, parsnip, Brussels sprouts, cabbage, lettuce, carrot, cauliflower, celery, collard greens, cucumber, fennel, kale, chayote , leeks, mushroom, asparagus, onion, okra, pumpkin, salad greens, squash, seaweed, spinach, sweet potato, turnip, zucchini, Swiss chard, watercress

Fruits – blackberry, banana, blueberry, guava, coconut, dates, grapes, grapefruit, kiwi, lemon, lychees, lime, melon, mango, orange, pears, papaya, peach, pineapple, pomegranate, raspberry, strawberry, watermelon

Meats – beef, chicken, pork, duck, turkey, rabbit, goat, bison, veal, quail, goose, elk, kangaroo, alligator, reindeer, moose, snake, pheasant, organ meats such as kidney, liver, heart, tongue, marrow and tripe

Herbs and Seasonings – garlic, onion powder, basil, bay leaves, ginger, cilantro, parsley, cinnamon, salt, peppermint, oregano, rosemary, thyme, turmeric, sage, horseradish, cloves, lemongrass, chamomile, edible flowers, coconut aminos, apple cider vinegar, balsamic vinegar, white vinegar

Seafood – tuna, red snapper, mackerel, salmon, tilapia, halibut, bass, sole, sardines, grouper, cod, clams, eel, crab, shrimp, anchovies, oysters, scallops, mussels, lobster, eel, mahi mahi, shark, abalone

Fermented food – coconut yoghurt, kombucha, kimchi, coconut kefir, sauerkraut

Healthy oils – coconut oil, olive oil, avocado oil, animal fat, lard, grass-fed ghee

Beverages – water, homemade fruit smoothies and vegetable shakes (omit nightshade vegetables), herbal teas

Other – homemade meat stock, canned coconut milk, coconut cream, honey, maples syrup, gelatin, arrowroot starch, coconut flour

Notes:

- Limit fruit intake to 20 grams per day;
- Check coconut products for gluten and other unhealthy chemicals;
- Choose vinegars that are sugar-free;
- Honey and maple syrup should be used in moderation; and
- Buy wild, grass-fed meat for healthier results.

Foods that are not allowed in the AIP diet:
Nightshade vegetables and spices – tomato, potato, eggplant, peppers, tomatillos, gooseberries, pepper flakes, cayenne pepper, chili pepper, paprika, garam masala powder, curry powder, hot sauce mixes

Dairy – eggs, mayonnaise, butter, soymilk, animal milk, sweetened condensed milk, ice cream, yoghurt, all-purpose cream, cheese

Legumes – red beans, lentils, garbanzo beans, snow peas, black beans, pinto beans, black eyed peas, mongo beans, soybeans, chickpeas, lima beans, kidney beans, tofu

Grains – wheat, rice, sorghum, oats, millet, corn, barley, spelt

Nuts and seeds – peanuts, quinoa, walnuts, chia seeds, pumpkin seeds, chestnuts, anise seed, cashews, sesame seeds, pecans, sunflower seeds, pistachios, hazelnuts, pine nuts, poppy seed, cumin, mustard seed, nutmeg, annatto seed, coriander, caraway, flax seeds

Processed food – pasta, cookies, pretzels, cakes, pancakes, waffles, chocolate bars, rice cakes, cold cuts, pizza, bread, potato chips, cereals

Beverages – brewed coffee, coffee blends, seed-based organic teas, soda, alcohol, milkshakes, sugar-rich teas, energy drinks

Other – sugars, algae, thickening agents, vegetable oils, seed-based oils, artificial seasonings, food additives, gluten-rich flours, dried fruit, vanilla

Foods prohibited in the AIP diet but can be reintroduced after the 30 days:
Egg yolks
Coffee
Nuts and seeds (including oils)
Small doses of gluten free alcohol
Chocolate
Paprika
Sweet Peppers
Eggplant

Notes:

- Reintroductions should only be made once autoimmune disease symptoms have significantly reduced;
- Once you are reintroducing foods, eat small amounts of an ingredient for 2-3 days;
- Look out for the following symptoms that imply food intolerance:
  - Worsening autoimmune disease symptoms
  - Fatigue
  - Headaches
  - Stomach problems
  - Muscle pain
  - Mood swings
  - Heightened food cravings

If you are feeling one of these symptoms, refrain from eating the food and stick to the AIP diet food list.

Now that you are aware of what to eat and which food items to avoid, it is now time to try the recipes in this book. This 7-day AIP meal plan is a well-balanced set of dishes that includes recipes for breakfast, lunch, dinner, snack, and dessert. It is expected that a one-week AIP diet trial will help control aggravating symptoms and revert the immune system to its healthy state.

Chapter 3: Day 1 of AIP Recipes

Brace yourself, for this is the start of a new day! The first day of an autoimmune paleo diet is never easy for unhealthy eaters like us. However, the key is to focus on the food list and try to get through the day without cheating on your diet.

Breakfast: Apple and Squash Morning Cereal

This heavenly paleo breakfast blends the naturally sweet flavors of coconut, apples and squash into one stomach-friendly meal. This is a healthier substitute for gluten rich oats and cereals.

Servings: 3
Cooking time: 15 minutes

Ingredients:
1 red apple, peeled, cored and grated
2 cups boiled butternut squash
4 tablespoons toasted coconut
1 cup organic coconut milk
½ teaspoon powdered ginger
1 teaspoon cinnamon powder

Pinch of salt

Instructions:

- Place the apple, butternut squash, coconut milk, ginger, cinnamon and salt in a blender and puree the ingredients for 30 seconds or until the desired consistency is reached.
- Pour the cereal mixture in a saucepan over medium flame and simmer it for 10 minutes.
- Place the cereal into individual bowls then sprinkle toasted coconut on top. Serve warm.

Snack: Vegetable Sticks and Beet Dip

Replace unhealthy potato chips and crackers with these crispy vegetable sticks dipped in a creamy roasted beet mixture.

Serves: 5
Cooking time: 1 hour 15 minutes

Ingredients:

1 cup celery sticks
1 cup cucumber sticks
1 cup carrot sticks
1 tablespoon melted coconut oil
1 kilogram beets, peeled and cubed
2 garlic cloves, peeled
1 tablespoon apple cider vinegar
3 tablespoons olive oil
2 teaspoons lemon juice
¼ cup water
Pinch of salt

Instructions:

- Preheat the oven to 375°F and prepare a heat-proof baking dish.
- Arrange the beets on the baking dish and drizzle the coconut oil on top.

- Place the dish in the oven and bake for 1 hour.
- Let the beets cool down for 10-15 minutes then place them in a blender together with the garlic, vinegar, olive oil, lemon juice, water and salt.
- Blend the dip mixture for 2 minutes then pour it in a bowl.
- Serve the beet dip with the celery, cucumber and carrot sticks.

Lunch: Seared Scallops with Spinach Puree

Complement those juicy, light scallops with blended greens that will help nourish the body and satisfy the taste buds.

Servings: 3
Cooking time: 40 minutes

Ingredients:
3 cups spinach, washed and drained
6 scallops
1 small radish, peeled and sliced
2 tablespoons coconut oil
1 tablespoon olive oil
Pinch of salt

Instructions:

- Place the sliced radish in a steamer and cook for 10 minutes.
- Once the radish is tender, place it in a food processor together with the spinach, salt and coconut oil.
- Pulse the radishes and spinach for 20 seconds and set it aside.
- Heat the olive oil in a pan over medium-high flame.

- Sear the sides of each scallop for 2-3 minutes.
- To assemble the dish, pour the spinach puree on the plate then place the seared scallops on top. Serve immediately.

Dinner: Zesty Broccoli Soup

Have a light and hearty vegetable soup for dinner to help cleanse your stomach and repair your body's cells as you go to sleep later in the evening.

Servings: 5
Cooking time: 10 minutes

Ingredients:
2 ½ cups broccoli florets, steamed
2 cups homemade chicken broth
3 teaspoons lemon juice
5 pieces basil leaves
1 tablespoon olive oil
Pinch of salt

Instructions:

- Mix together the broccoli, broth, lemon juice, basil, olive oil and salt in a food processer.
- Process the ingredients for 2-3 minutes.
- Pour the soup in a saucepan and simmer for 5 minutes before serving.

Dessert: Blackberry Lime Pastry

Replace that sinful slice of blueberry cheesecake with this scrumptious gluten free dessert that will satisfy your sweet tooth.

Serves: 6
Cooking time: 2 hours

Ingredients:
8 cups blackberries, washed and drained
2 cups sweet potato flour
3 tablespoons lime juice
2 tablespoons honey
½ teaspoon salt
½ cup olive oil
1 can chilled coconut milk
1 teaspoon lime zest
Pinch of salt

Instructions:

- Preheat the oven to 350°F and prepare a round pie dish.
- Place the blackberries, lime juice and honey in a pot over medium flame and simmer for 1 hour.
- While the berries are cooking, place the flour, salt, lime zest and oil in a blender and mix for 1-2 minutes.

- Once the dough is wet, press it down the pie dish and evenly spread it towards the sides.
- Place the crust in the oven and bake for 20 minutes.
- Remove the baked crust from the oven and let it cool completely.
- After an hour of simmering the berries, pour the mixture into a bowl through a strainer.
- Place the strained blackberries on the baked crust and spread evenly.
- Chill the pastry in the fridge for 1 hour.
- Spoon the solidified coconut milk from the can and place it in a bowl. Whisk it for 2-3 minutes to produce coconut cream.
- Take out the chilled pastry and cut into 6 equal slices. Spoon a portion of the coconut cream on top of each slice before serving.

Chapter 4: Day 2 of AIP Recipes

If Day 1 under the AIP diet was difficult, today may be a bit more stressful as you have already realized how drastic this lifestyle change is in terms of having limited food choices. Fortunately, the following recipes will help you cope with the change by greatly satisfying your taste buds.

Breakfast: Coconut Lychee Cereal

Lychees are small, delectable fruits found in Asian food shops that add a sweet and refreshing flavor profile to coconut dishes.

Serves: 3
Cooking time: 25 minutes

Ingredients:
5 lychees, peeled, pitted and chopped
2 cups coconut flakes
1 cup coconut milk
1 tablespoon coconut manna, melted
½ teaspoon cinnamon powder
1 tablespoon coconut oil, melted
1 teaspoon lemon zest
Pinch of salt

Instructions:

- Get a small mixing bowl and blend together the coconut manna, coconut oil and cinnamon powder.
- Add in the lemon zest, salt and coconut flakes then toss.
- Place the seasoned coconut flakes on a baking sheet and place it in a 325°F oven.
- Bake the flakes for 12 minutes or until it turns golden brown.
- Place the coconut flakes in a serving bowl then mix in the lychee and coconut milk. Serve immediately.

Snack: Garlic-roasted Cauliflower Bites

Savor the rich aroma of this oven-roasted vegetable snack which blends the clean flavors of cauliflower with the pungent zest of garlic.

Serves: 3
Cooking time: 1 hour 30 minutes

Ingredients:

1 medium head of cauliflower, trimmed
1 tablespoon chopped fresh thyme
4 garlic cloves, minced
2 tablespoons coconut oil
Pinch of sea salt

Instructions:

- Heat the coconut oil in a pan over medium heat.
- Add in the garlic and thyme and cook for 1 minute.
- Place the cauliflower on a baking dish then pour the garlic and thyme infusion all over the vegetable.
- Sprinkle sea salt on top of the cauliflower.
- Bake the cauliflower in the oven for 1 hour and 15 minutes or until it becomes tender.

The cauliflower is ready once you are able to insert a knife through it easily.

- Break the cauliflower into florets and let it cool before placing in an airtight container.

Lunch: Paleo Fruity Steak Salad

This lunch recipe is a wonderful balance of protein, vegetables and healthy fats that help fill the stomach and provide mid-day energy.

Serves: 3
Cooking time: 30 minutes

Ingredients:
3 pieces 150-gram steaks
2 peaches, pitted and cubed
1 head iceberg lettuce, chopped
1 tablespoon apple cider vinegar
3 tablespoons olive oil

Instructions:

- Sear each side of the steak for 10 minutes.
- Once the meat is cooked, chop the steak into bite-size pieces.
- Get a salad bowl and whisk together the vinegar and olive oil.
- Blend in the lettuce, chopped steak and cubed peaches then toss.
- Serve the salad warm or cold.

Dinner: Avocado Bacon Cups

Who says bacon is just for breakfast? This dinner recipe proves that the crisp, meaty flavors of bacon can be an early evening treat most especially if it is combined with the zesty flavors of avocado and lime.

Serves: 3 (2 bacon cups/serving)
Cooking time: 40 minutes

Ingredients:
18 pieces thin bacon slices, sliced as needed
1 avocado, peeled, pitted and diced
2 teaspoons fresh lime juice
½ cup chopped fresh parsley

Instructions:

- Mix together the avocado, lime juice and parsley in a bowl and set it aside.
- Turn over a muffin tin. Use 3 bacon slices to wrap each cup (1 ½ slice around the sides then 1 ½ slice to cover the base of the cup).
- Place the muffin tin on a larger baking sheet for it to catch the bacon drippings.
- Bake the bacon cups in a 350°F oven for 20 minutes or until the bacon is crisp.
- Cool the bacon cups in room temperature for 5 minutes.

- Spoon the avocado mixture into the cups. Serve immediately.

Dessert: Apple Pie

This delectable dessert uses autoimmune paleo-friendly flours such as arrowroot starch and coconut flour to create a healthier version of a favorite dessert.

Serves: 6
Cooking time: 1 hour

Ingredients:

3 red apples, peeled, cored and sliced
2 tablespoons lemon juice
1 teaspoon cinnamon
2 tablespoons honey
1 cup arrowroot starch
1 cup coconut flour
½ cup cold water
¾ cup coconut oil
Pinch of sea salt

Instructions:

- Preheat the oven to 350°F and prepare a 9-inch pie plate.
- Mix the arrowroot starch, coconut flour and salt in a large bowl.
- Blend in the coconut oil into the dry ingredients by cutting it into the flour with a pastry cutter.

- Slowly pour the water into the dry ingredients and knead it until the dough becomes moist yet crumbly.
- Press the dough into the pie plate and poke a few holes on the base with a fork.
- Bake the pie crust in the oven for 20 minutes.
- While the pie crust is baking, place the apples, lemon juice, cinnamon and honey in a saucepan and simmer for 20 minutes or until the apples are tender.
- Take out the pie crust then pour in the apple mixture. Place the pie back in the oven and bake for another 10 minutes.
- Slice the pie into 6 equal portions before serving.

Chapter 5: Day 3 of AIP Recipes

This revamped version of the Paleolithic diet may be stirring up your curiosity by now because the first few days under the AIP lifestyle made you realize that clean eating can be deliciously satisfying. Try out the recipes in this chapter and delight yourself with the clean flavors of each dish.

Breakfast: Herbed Breakfast Sausages

Grass-fed beef is the best option to make a nutritious and tasty breakfast sausage, but you can reinvent this recipe with ground chicken or flaked fish for a lighter morning meal.

Serves: 2
Cooking time: 30 minutes

Ingredients:
500 grams ground beef
½ teaspoon garlic powder
½ teaspoon onion powder
1 tablespoon chopped cilantro
5 basil leaves, chopped
2 tablespoons olive oil
½ teaspoon sea salt

Instructions:

- Mix the beef, cilantro, salt, garlic powder, onion powder, basil and sea salt in a bowl until the ingredients are well-incorporated.
- Form the sausage mixture into 4 patties.
- Heat the olive oil in a large pan over medium-high flame.
- Cook each side of the patty for 8-10 minutes or until it becomes golden brown. Serve while hot.

Snack: Ginger Mango Smoothie

Enjoy the freshness of this organic brew that's low in sugar but high in gut-soothing properties.

Serves: 2
Cooking time: 10 minutes

Ingredients:
1-inch ginger, peeled
3 cups cubed ripe mango
1 cucumber, peeled and diced
1 cup chopped celery
Juice from 1 orange
2 cups water
1 cup chopped parsley

Instructions:

- Place celery, parsley and water in a blender and pulse for 3-5 times.
- Add in the ginger, mango, cucumber and orange juice and blend for 2-3 minutes.
- Pour the smoothie in a glass and serve.

Lunch: Sautéed Brussels Sprout

This vegetable dish is so easy to make, you can cook it ahead of time and place it in the fridge for a healthy mid-day meal you can bring with you to the office.

Serves: 2
Cooking time: 30 minutes

Ingredients:

1 kilogram Brussels sprouts, trimmed and halved
Pinch of sea salt
2 teaspoons fresh lemon juice
300 grams bacon, chopped

Instructions:

- Place the Brussels sprouts in a pot filled with water and boil it over medium-high flame for 10 minutes.
- After 10 minutes, turn off the heat and drain the cooked vegetables.
- Brown the bacon pieces in a large skillet over medium-high flame.
- Once the bacon is crispy, mix in the vegetables and salt and cook for 10 minutes.
- Sprinkle the lemon juice on top of the sautéed vegetables and toss before serving.

Dinner: Creamy Green Chowder

Green leafy vegetables, such as kale and spinach, are the most vitamin-packed ingredients you can use to whip up a gut-friendly AIP dinner. Add in some herbs and coconut cream and you have a scrumptious meal that even the kids will love.

Serves: 2
Cooking time: 40 minutes

Ingredients:
4 tablespoons coconut cream
3 cups chicken broth
2 garlic cloves, minced
4 thyme sprigs, chopped
6 cups chopped kale leaves
3 cups chopped okra
1 cup chopped spinach leaves
1 cup water

Instructions:
- Place a large pot over medium-high flame.
- Add in the chicken broth, water, garlic, thyme, kale, okra and spinach to the pot and mix well.
- Cover the pot and simmer the ingredients for 25 minutes.

- Transfer the contents of the pot into a blender.
- Pour the coconut cream into the blender and puree the chowder for 2 minutes.
- Pour the dish in individual bowls and serve immediately. You may also place it in a mason jar and keep it in the fridge for 2-3 days.

Dessert: Mango Jelly Bites

It is recommended that you make extra batches of these jelly bites because the whole family will definitely love biting into these sweet and healthy treats.

Serves: 6 servings (4 gummies/serving)
Preparation time: 1 hour 15 minutes

Ingredients:
1 ½ cup chopped ripe mangoes
¾ cup fresh lemon juice
¼ cup of grass-fed gelatin
2 tablespoons honey

Instructions:

- Place lemon juice and chopped mangoes in a blender and puree them for 1 minute.
- Pour the mango puree in a saucepan then add in the honey and gelatin.
- Turn the flame to low and cook the mixture for 5-7 minutes while constantly stirring it.
- Spoon the jelly into a rectangular baking pan and place it in the fridge for 1 hour.
- Once the jelly is set, cut it into 24 even slices and remove it from the pan before serving.

Chapter 6: Day 4 of AIP Recipes

If you are feeling a bit lighter and notice that small aches and pains have disappeared, it is because your body is slowly becoming free from the toxins and bacteria of processed food. Just keep on walking towards better health by cooking these flavorful AIP dishes.

Breakfast: Cinnamon Banana Pancakes

These dairy-free and egg-free pancakes are not only delicious, but they are full of calcium, good fats and potassium that are healing to the body.

Serves: 2
Cooking time: 30 minutes

Ingredients:
4 overripe bananas, mashed
2 tablespoons coconut oil
½ teaspoon cinnamon powder
½ teaspoon allspice
2 tablespoons maple syrup

Instructions:

- Mix the mashed banana, cinnamon and allspice in a bowl. Set these aside.
- Heat the coconut oil on a pan over medium flame.
- Place spoonfuls of the pancake batter onto the pan and cook for 8 minutes.
- Flip the pancake over and cook the other side for another 8 minutes.
- Place the pancakes on a serving plate and drizzle the maple syrup on top before serving.

Snack: Vitamin Chips

Craving for something salty and crisp? Try this healthy vegetable chip recipe that is full of fiber, calcium and other vitamins that fend off disease and prevent aggravating aches and pains.

Serves: 5
Cooking time: 30 minutes

Ingredients:
8 cups kale leaves, torn and washed
½ teaspoon sea salt
3 tablespoons coconut oil, melted

Instructions:

- Preheat the oven to 350°F and prepare a parchment-lined baking sheet.
- Dry the kale leaves with a paper towel and place them in a bowl.
- Pour the coconut oil over the kale leaves then sprinkle sea salt on top.
- Toss the kale until the leaves are evenly coated with oil and salt.
- Place the kale leaves on the baking sheet and bake it in the oven for 20 minutes. Serve immediately.

Lunch: Paleo Spaghetti with Meatballs

A refreshing take on a kid's favorite, this autoimmune paleo-friendly dish will surprise and delight the family with its savory flavors.

Serves: 4
Cooking time: 45 minutes

Ingredients:
800 grams ground beef
1 cup fresh basil, chopped
Pinch of salt
1 kilogram zucchini
5 slices bacon, chopped
10 garlic cloves, minced
1 ¼ cup button mushrooms, sliced
1 cup black olives, pitted and sliced

Instructions:

- Line a baking sheet with parchment and preheat the oven to 400°F.
- To make the meatballs, combine the beef, ¼ cup basil and salt in a bowl.
- Form 20 meatballs from the mixture and place it on the lined baking sheet.
- Bake the meatballs in the oven for 15 minutes.

- To make the noodles, place the zucchini through a spiral cutter or slice it into thin, pasta-like strips.
- Place the zucchini pasta in a colander and sprinkle with salt.
- Leave it standing for an hour to allow the water to drain off of the zucchini.
- After an hour, rinse the zucchini noodles and dry them completely with a paper towel.
- Place a large pan over medium flame then add in the bacon slices. Cook it for 7 minutes.
- Blend in the mushrooms, garlic and olives and sauté for another 7 minutes.
- Pour the zucchini noodles into the pan then add the basil.
- Toss the noodles for 5 minutes then add the baked meatballs. Serve warm.

Dinner: Chunky Cauliflower Soup

If you want to have a low-carbohydrate AIP dish for dinner, try this flavorful soup recipe that will make you appreciate the fact that you have gone into an organic lifestyle of eating.

Serves: 2
Cooking time: 45 minutes

Ingredients:
4 cups homemade chicken stock
1 kilogram cauliflower florets, chopped
2 leeks, sliced
½ cup chopped fresh parsley
3 bacon slices, chopped
2 garlic cloves, crushed
½ teaspoon powdered ginger
1 tablespoon white vinegar
Pinch of salt

Instructions:

- Place the bacon in a large pot and let it brown over medium-high heat.
- Remove the cooked bacon from the pot and set it aside.
- Add the garlic, powdered ginger and leeks in the pot and cook for 3 minutes.

- Mix in the cauliflower, salt, vinegar and broth then cover the pot.
- Simmer the soup for 10 minutes.
- Turn off the heat then transfer the contents of the pot to a blender.
- Process the hot soup for 2 minutes then pour it in a serving bowl.
- Sprinkle the parsley and bacon on top of each soup bowl before serving.

Dessert: Pumpkin Apple Parfait

Enjoy delectable layers of pumpkin, apples and coconut in one immune-boosting jar of dessert.

Serves: 2
Cooking time: 1 hour 15 minutes

Ingredients:

4 cups cooked pumpkin, pureed
2 cups pureed apples
1 can coconut milk
1 cup toasted coconut flakes
1 teaspoon cinnamon
1 teaspoon honey
Pinch of salt
1 teaspoon powdered ginger

Instructions:

- Place the pumpkin puree in a saucepan over medium flame.
- Mix in the cinnamon, honey, salt and ginger and heat it for 1-2 minutes. Set this aside.
- Scoop out the solidified portion of the coconut milk and place it in a bowl. Whisk the coconut milk for 2 minutes until a creamy mixture is produced.

- To assemble the dessert, prepare a mason jar and place 3 tablespoons of the pumpkin puree at the bottom.
- Spoon 2 tablespoons of the apple puree on top of the pumpkin, followed by 2 tablespoons of the whipped coconut cream.
- Sprinkle ¼ cup of the coconut flakes on top of the cream. Repeat the layering and do the same method for the remaining ingredients.
- Chill the dessert in the fridge for at least one hour. Serve cold.

Chapter 7: Day 5 of AIP Recipes

By now, you have probably gotten used to eating healthy and may have small cravings for chocolate or cheese. Going on the AIP diet requires 100% commitment, so keep yourself focused and remember that the path you are taking will lead you to a healthier, pain-free life.

Breakfast: Collard Greens and Carrots Stir Fry

This stir fry recipe is a great way to mix vegetables, protein and healthy fats into one immunity-boosting plate.

Serves: 2
Cooking time: 30 minutes

Ingredients:
2 cups chopped collard greens
1 large carrot, peeled and sliced
2 garlic cloves, crushed
1 teaspoon onion powder
½ cup mushrooms, sliced
½ cup chopped cauliflower
1 tablespoon coconut oil

1 teaspoon lime juice
Pinch of sea salt

Instructions:

- Heat the oil in a pan over medium-high flame.
- Add in the garlic, onion powder and carrots and cook for 15 minutes.
- Once the carrots are tender, add the mushrooms and cauliflower to the pan and cook for 5 minutes.
- Mix in the collard greens, lime juice and salt.
- Stir-fry the dish for 5 minutes or until the greens have wilted. Place it in a bowl and serve immediately.

Snack: Banana Crisps

Satisfy your midday sweet cravings by munching on these dairy-free and gut-friendly fruit crackers. They taste better than cookies and respond well with the body's hormones.

Serves: 2
Cooking time: 1 hour 15 minutes

Ingredients:
½ cup extra virgin coconut oil
Pinch of salt
2 large ripe bananas

Instructions:

- Preheat the oven to 325°F and line a baking sheet with parchment.
- Place the bananas, oil and salt in a blender and process for 4 minutes.
- Pour the banana batter on the baking sheet.
- Use a spatula to spread the batter outwards until it becomes a thin layer over the parchment.
- Bake the batter for 10 minutes in the oven.
- After 10 minutes, take out the baking sheet and score the banana batter with a pizza cutter to form squares.

- Place the sheet back in the oven and bake it for 1 hour.
- Break apart the cracker and place it on a wire rack to cool.

Lunch: Tangy Summer Squash Soup

This thick and creamy soup is a great working lunch dish: just pour it in a mason jar, chill it in the fridge and grab it from the kitchen before leaving for work.

Serves: 2
Cooking time: 20 minutes

Ingredients:
2½ cups cubed summer squash, peeled
½ cup homemade chicken stock
2 teaspoons lime juice
2 teaspoons apple cider vinegar
1 teaspoon lime zest
1 cup chopped white onion
3 tablespoons olive oil
Pinch of sea salt

Instructions:

- Heat a tablespoon of the olive oil in a large pan over medium flame.
- Add the squash and onions to the pan and sauté for 5 minutes.
- Pour in the vinegar and simmer the squash for 15 minutes.

- Transfer the contents of the pan into a blender then mix in the stock, lime juice, lime zest, onion, olive oil and salt.
- Cover the blender then puree the soup for 2 minutes.
- Serve the soup immediately or let it cool down before pouring it into mason jars for storage in the fridge.

Dinner: Grilled Salmon with Avocado Thyme Dressing

Savor this light, delicious entrée filled with vitamins and omega 3 fatty acids that help maintain a healthy immune system.

Serves: 3
Cooking time: 45 minutes

Ingredients:
2 tablespoons coconut oil
3 salmon fillets
2 garlic cloves, crushed
1 tablespoon lemon zest
1 teaspoon capers
1 ripe avocado, peeled and pitted
½ cup chopped thyme

Instructions:

- In a small bowl, mash the avocado together with the garlic, thyme, capers and zest. Mix well and set aside.
- Grease the grill pan with a third of the coconut oil and place it over medium-high heat.
- Place the salmon fillet on the grill pan with the skin side up. Grill for 8 minutes.

- Flip the salmon over and cook the skin for 4 minutes. Do the same process for the remaining fillets.
- Place the fillets on a serving platter. Spoon the avocado and thyme dressing on the side of the fish and serve.

Dessert: Mixed Berries Cobbler

Satisfy your sweet tooth with a slice of this scrumptious cobbler that is free of gluten, dairy and refined sugars that may affect one's hormones.

Serves: 8
Cooking time: 45 minutes

Ingredients:

¾ cup blueberries, washed and drained
¾ cup raspberries, washed and drained
3 tablespoons water
2 teaspoons lemon juice
2 ½ tablespoons coconut oil
½ cup arrowroot flour
¾ cup baking soda
3 tablespoons honey
¼ teaspoon salt

Instructions:

- Grease an 8-inch ceramic oven dish with ½ tablespoon coconut oil and preheat the oven to 325°F.
- Arrange the blueberries and raspberries at the bottom of the dish. Set this aside.

- Place the water, lemon juice, flour, baking soda, honey, salt and the remaining coconut oil in a bowl and mix well.
- Spread the flour mixture over the berries.
- Bake the cobbler for 30-35 minutes. Serve warm.

Chapter 8: Day 6 of AIP Recipes

If you have not strayed from the AIP meal plan, give yourself a pat on the back. You are on the 6th day of healing your gut with food, and what better way to celebrate better health than by preparing organic, stomach-friendly meals for you and the family.

Breakfast: Minty Morning Grapefruit Salad

Start off the day with a refreshingly sweet and minty blend of fruits and herbs that will help regulate digestion throughout the day.

Serves: 4
Cooking time: 10 minutes

Ingredients:
7 fresh mint leaves, chopped
3 pink grapefruits, peeled, pitted and sliced into thin segments
2 small apples, cored and sliced into thin segments
½ cup lemon juice
1 tablespoon honey
¼ teaspoon sea salt

Instructions:

- Place the grapefruit, apple, lemon juice and honey in a salad bowl and toss.
- Sprinkle salt and mint leaves on top before serving.

Snack: Homemade Beef Jerky

Place a couple of these beef munchies in an airtight container and put it in a child-friendly area in the kitchen: the little ones will certainly love snacking on this meaty treat.

Serves: 4
Cooking time: 8 hours 15 minutes

Ingredients:
500 grams grass fed beef roast
2 tablespoons sea salt

Instructions:

- Use a sharp knife to cut the beef into thin slices.
- Mix the beef slices and sea salt in a bowl.
- Skewer the tips of the beef strips through wooden sticks and arrange them evenly beside one another.
- Place the skewers in the oven and allow the beef strips to hang through the oven rack.
- Set the oven temperature to 200°F.
- Place a wooden spoon on the oven door to allow some moisture to escape from inside the oven.
- Cook the beef jerky for 8 hours. Let it cool completely before storing it.

Lunch: *Yummy Sweet Potato and Carrot Soup*

This flavorful AIP-friendly soup is a great freezer meal that you can store in a mason jar and heat in the microwave just in time for lunch.

Serves: 3
Cooking time: 40 minutes

Ingredients:
4 sweet potatoes, peeled and diced
1 yellow onion, minced
3 small carrots, peeled and diced
1 pear, peeled, cored and diced
4 cups homemade chicken stock
Pinch of salt

Instructions:

- Place a large pot over medium-high flame.
- Place the potatoes, carrots, pears, onion, salt and stock in the pot and cover it. Boil the ingredients for 30 minutes.
- Uncover the pot and turn off the burner.
- Using an immersion blender, puree the soup until a smooth texture is produced.
- Ladle the soup into bowls or mason jars and serve.

Dinner: Chicken and Cauliflower Rice Bowl

If you are strictly following the AIP diet and have a sudden craving for rice, try this dinner recipe which uses cauliflower as a filling and delicious rice substitute.

Serves: 3
Cooking time: 40 minutes

Ingredients:

3 cups cauliflower florets
3 cooked chicken breasts, shredded
1 tablespoon coconut aminos
2 garlic cloves, crushed
1 tablespoon chopped fresh ginger
2 tablespoons olive oil
Pinch of salt
½ teaspoon dried rosemary
1 tablespoon parsley

Instructions:

- Process all the cauliflower florets in a blender for 1 minute. Do this in 2-3 batches until a textured, rice-like consistency is reached.
- Heat the olive oil in a large pan over medium-high flame.

- Add in the garlic, ginger, rosemary and sauté for 3 minutes.
- Mix in the cauliflower rice and cook for 5-10 minutes.
- Once the cauliflower is tender, add in the shredded chicken, coconut aminos, salt and parsley.
- Keep sautéing the dish for 2-3 minutes then turn off the heat. Serve the rice warm in individual bowls.

Dessert: Raspberry Coconut Mousse

This sweet and creamy mousse is the perfect dessert to cap off a stressful day. It's light, fruity and contains a glass-full of immunity-boosting nutrients.

Serves: 3
Cooking time: 2 hours 5 minutes

Ingredients:
2 cups raspberries, washed and drained
2 tablespoons maple syrup
1 ½ tablespoon apple cider vinegar
½ cup coconut flakes
1 tablespoon grass-fed gelatin
1 ½ cup organic coconut milk
½ teaspoon lemon juice

Instructions:

- Place the raspberries, maple syrup, vinegar, coconut flakes, gelatin, coconut milk and lemon juice in a blender and process it for 1-2 minutes.
- Scoop the mousse into individual jars or glasses and chill in the fridge for 2 hours before serving.

Chapter 9: Day 7 of AIP Recipes

Congratulations! You are on your 7th day under the AIP diet plan. By now, you have successfully learned how to cook healthier meals that will help lessen the chances of having full-blown autoimmune disease.

Since you have lasted this long in the AIP journey and have had positive changes in your digestion, why not adopt this positive lifestyle change for the long haul?

Breakfast: Banana, Berry and Spinach Smoothie

This breakfast smoothie is packed with nutrients and flavors that will help rev up your body's energy in the morning.

Serves: 2
Cooking time: 1 hour 5 minutes

Ingredients:
½ cup blueberries
½ cup strawberries
2 bananas, chopped
1½ cups chopped spinach
1 cup water

½ cup fresh orange juice

Instructions:

- Place the blueberries, strawberries, chopped bananas, spinach, orange juice and water in a blender and process it for 2 minutes.
- Pour the smoothie in individual glasses and chill in the fridge for 1 hour before serving.

Snack: Grain-Free Garlic Breadsticks

This dairy-free breadstick recipe is a delicious blend of AIP-friendly flours, herbs and seasonings, thus making it a perfect snack for people with autoimmune symptoms.

Serves: 4
Cooking time: 15 minutes

Ingredients:
1/3 cup arrowroot starch
½ teaspoon baking soda
1/3 cup coconut flour
1 teaspoon fresh rosemary
3 tablespoons water
2 teaspoons lemon juice
1 tablespoon gelatin, dissolved in 3 tablespoons water
4 tablespoons olive oil
Pinch of sea salt
Pinch of garlic powder

Instructions:

- Preheat the oven to 350°F and prepare a parchment-lined baking sheet.
- Prepare the egg substitute by placing the dissolved gelatin in a bowl. Pour in boiling

hot water and whisk the mixture until a thick paste forms. Set this aside.

- Mix together the arrowroot starch, coconut flour, rosemary, lemon juice, and 3 tablespoons of the olive oil.
- Blend the egg substitute into the flour mixture and knead it until the dough is formed.
- Divide the dough into 8 equal-sized balls and roll each ball into long breadsticks.
- Place the breadsticks on the baking sheet and brush it with the remaining olive oil.
- Sprinkle the salt and garlic powder on top of the breadsticks.
- Bake the breadsticks in the oven for 12 minutes. Let it cool before serving.

Lunch: Garlic Chicken with Fennel and Carrots

This chicken recipe is usually served with rice, but AIP advocates can eat this entrée on its own and still be satisfied by its aromatic flavors.

Serves: 3
Cooking time: 20 minutes

Ingredients:
3 boneless chicken breasts
3 teaspoons garlic powder
Pinch of salt
2 tablespoons olive oil
½ fennel bulb, trimmed and sliced thinly
2 carrots, peeled and sliced into thin quarters
½ cup pitted black olives, sliced
½ cup fresh orange juice
½ cup chopped ripe mangoes
½ cup homemade chicken broth

Instructions:

- In a small bowl, place the chicken breasts and rub it with garlic powder and salt. Set this aside.

- Heat the oil in a large skillet over medium-high heat and place the chicken breasts on the pan.
- Cook each side of the chicken breast for 3 minutes.
- Transfer the cooked chicken breasts to a plate and set them aside.
- Place the carrots and fennel into the skillet and cook for 7 minutes.
- Add in the olives, mangoes, orange juice, chicken broth and chicken breasts and simmer the dish for 15 minutes. Serve immediately.

Dinner: Paleo Seafood Chowder

Warm up the cold nights with this hearty, gluten free chowder that combines leafy greens with nutritious meat from the sea.

Serves: 2
Cooking time: 15 minutes

Ingredients:
2 cups homemade chicken stock
½ cup chopped collard greens
1 cup chopped cabbage
5 mushrooms, sliced
5 prawns, peeled and deveined
2 cream dory fillets, sliced into chunks
1 cup coconut cream
Pinch of salt

Instructions:

- Pour the chicken stock in a large pot over medium-high flame and allow it to boil.
- Once the stock is boiling, mix in the collard greens, cabbage and mushrooms. Cook the vegetables for 10 minutes.
- Mix in the prawns, cream dory and salt. Boil the ingredients for 5-10 minutes.
- Pour in the coconut cream then lower the heat.

- Simmer the chowder for 8 minutes. Serve immediately.

Dessert: Lemon-Drizzled Papaya

Papaya is a flavorful tropical fruit that contains high doses of fiber, potassium and Vitamin C, hence making an effective immunity booster.

Serves: 2
Cooking time: 10 minutes

Ingredients:

1 solo papaya, peeled
2 tablespoons fresh lemon juice
½ teaspoon honey

Instructions:

- Slice the papaya in half and scoop out the seeds.
- Cut the fruit into wedges and place it in a serving platter.
- Drizzle the honey and lemon juice over the wedges and serve. You can likewise chill the fruit for 1 hour before serving.

Chapter 10: Eight Tips to Keep You on Track with The Autoimmune Paleo Diet

"I try to focus on the fact that that I have a strategy for improving my health that is far more powerful than any prescription medication."

Sarah Ballantyne, PhD
Author, *The Paleo Approach*

If you are ready to try the autoimmune paleo diet but feel a bit anxious about its food restrictions, or if you have been practicing this organic lifestyle but feel compelled to revert back to your old ways because of food cravings, do not lose hope. There are simple techniques that will help you stick to this life-changing diet and potentially heal your body for life.

Here are eight tips to help keep you on track with the AIP diet:

1. *Keep an AIP food journal*
   One of the best ways to stick to a new routine is to journal your activities. Jotting down important details of your daily life

such as the AIP meals you have eaten, specific aches, allergic reactions to food and emotional ups and downs will help motivate you and build your commitment towards recovery from autoimmunity.

Write down your AIP-related experiences in a journal. Feel free to express your innermost feelings and thoughts: this is an effective way to document the whole AIP process most especially when you start re-introducing other foods into your system. In addition, your journal will serve as proof of your AIP progression and will motivate you to push even further.

2. *Do extensive research on the AIP diet*
   Before starting on this new life towards self-healing, do a complete research on autoimmune diseases as well as the guidelines of autoimmune paleo meal planning. Reading on these facts will help you ascertain if changing to an AIP lifestyle will address your recent health concerns.

   Luckily, there are a lot of websites on the internet that are solely dedicated to teaching people about the benefits of the autoimmune paleo diet and provide links to books, recipes, AIP nutritionists and other valuable readings. Equip yourself with enough information that will help you commit to this drastic lifestyle change.

3. *Plan your weekly meals*
   If you want to try the AIP diet, follow the 7-day sample meal plan provided in this book. The recipes include dishes for breakfast, lunch, dinner, snack and dessert which serve as a complete guide in your week-long meal preparation. The AIP meal plan teaches you simple ways to cook gut-friendly dishes and equip you with the right tools to begin your journey towards wellness.

   Meal planning may prove to be challenging, but it is an important factor in surviving the AIP diet. Allow yourself to be guided by the AIP food list while creating delectable dishes for you and your family. This habit will protect you from falling into temptation or straying from the diet's guidelines.

4. *Shop for ingredients that are allowed in the AIP food list*
   If you have read the 2nd chapter of this book, you will find that the AIP food list

includes a rich variety of fresh ingredients that will help you prepare appetizing dishes. The key is to make the AIP food list your checklist whenever you take a trip to the market or grocery.

To ensure that you reap the benefits of a nutritious and cell-building AIP lifestyle, buy produce from the outer aisles of the grocery, specifically in the meat, vegetables, seafood and fruit sections. You can check the other lanes and shop for healthy oils and gluten free flours, but make sure to stay away from products that are refined, processed and prohibited in the AIP food list.

5. *Pack your own lunches*
   There will be days that co-workers will ask you to join them for lunch at the office cafeteria or for a late afternoon coffee break at Starbucks. How do you handle these temptations? Simply say no.

   Embracing an AIP lifestyle entails 100% commitment to its guidelines and recipes. There is no room for cheating as that will just slow down your recovery. That is why it is recommended that you cook your own

AIP-friendly meals and bring them with you to school or work. Who knows, you may even influence a co-worker to join you in your journey towards optimal wellness.

6. Tell your family and friends about your lifestyle change
   Family dinners and weekend lunches can be somewhat gut-wrenching for autoimmune disease sufferers, literally and figuratively. Aside from being tempted by an array of delectable grains, fried entrees and mouth-watering desserts, some family members may be appalled by your food restrictions and would even try to discourage you from continuing the AIP lifestyle.

   As soon as a loved one notices your self-imposed food restrictions during parties, explain to them the benefits of the AIP diet including how it is helping you regain control over your health. This will help them understand your organic food choices and realize that they too will greatly benefit from a Paleolithic diet.

7. Choose a credible AIP-specialized nutritionist

While doing research on the autoimmune paleo diet, check the internet for a list of licensed AIP nutritionists within your area. An autoimmune disease is a debilitating chronic illness that needs to be addressed immediately, and the smartest way to start the healing process is to look for an AIP expert you can trust your life with.

Make several calls and inquiries with AIP advocates and autoimmune disease support groups to help you look for a reputable nutritionist who specializes in AIP meal planning. Set up a meeting with him/ her then ask questions related to AIP and your health. Develop a healthy bond with your nutritionist so he/ she can help you manage autoimmune disease through proper nutrition.

8. *Make positive changes to other aspects of your life*
   This informative book provides sample recipes that will help you eat cleaner, gut-friendly food. However, there are other habits that need to be tweaked in order to heal autoimmune disease. Try making light, positive changes to your sleeping patterns, exercise routines and stress relief activities.

These factors should go hand-in-hand with proper nutrition in order to have a healthy and well-balanced life.

The AIP diet is more than just a spin-off of the paleo diet: it is a lifestyle change that leads you towards increased health awareness and pushes you towards cleaner eating habits. All these efforts are geared towards healing the body and eliminating the symptoms of autoimmune disease.

If you or a loved one has exhibited signs of having an autoimmune disease, start the AIP diet now so you can start flushing away the pains and rebuilding your health. We are only given one chance at living, so let's choose to lead a happier and disease-free life by eating healthier.

Conclusion

Thank you again for buying this book!

I hope this book was able to help you cook deliciously healthy autoimmune paleo dishes by following the sample 7-day meal plan that includes a vast array of immunity-boosting ingredients.

It is expected that upon reading this book, people who are suffering from autoimmune disease or are showing early signs of chronic illness will be enlightened by the fact that food can be an effective treatment of gut problems provided that we follow an organic diet that is free of sugar, dairy, gluten and other stomach-reactive foods.

The next step is to fill up your pantry with ingredients found in the AIP diet food list so you can try out other gut-friendly recipes that are available in paleo books and AIP websites.

Finally, if you enjoyed this book, please take the time to share your thoughts and post a review on Amazon. It'd be greatly appreciated!

Thank you and good luck!

Made in the USA
San Bernardino, CA
08 July 2015